MICROCOSM · PUBLISHING

Microcosm is Portland's autistic-founded, worker-owned, and most diversified publishing house and distributor with a focus on the colorful, authentic, and empowering. Our books and zines have put your power in your hands since 1996, equipping readers to make positive changes in their lives and in the world around them. Microcosm emphasizes skill-building, showing hidden histories, and fostering creativity through challenging conventional publishing wisdom with books and bookettes about DIY skills, food, bicycling, gender, self-care, and social justice.

Perfect Mix Tape Segue #3: 'fixing the plumbing'

About three or four years ago I thought that I quit making zines. I was done. I thought other people could spell out my thoughts and feelings better than I could. I preferred to read someone else's words and say 'fuck yea!' when that person really struck a chord with me.

Of course a zine maker can never really quit making zines. There's a sinking, internal need that creeps up now and again to purge yourself of your thoughts and make them public. Some people take years off in between issues or switch to related projects or write about their thoughts on the internet, but I hate that shit. I still had a bit of the zine bug in me when my friends started encouraging me to write zines about issues I was facing and discussing related issues.

That's the reason that I've made my last 4 zines and this one is no different.

It may read like a sob story but it's really just to clear some shit up and purify it from myself. I'm not looking for condolences or I'm sorrys. Most of this shit is dealt with. That's the only reason that I'm able to be writing about it now.

Thanks! Keep it real..

Joe

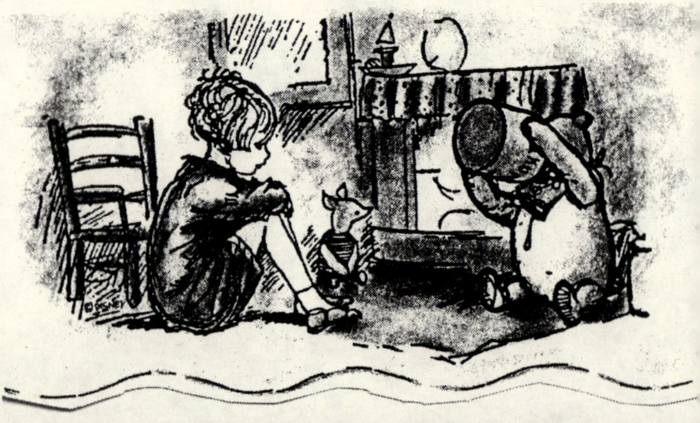

started about 6 years ago. Most of my old riends began to have accidental children. irst it seemed like one isolated incident fter another and then it started to seem ike everyone was having babies. This trend as only picked up as time goes by.

All of these accidental babies started to become really distressing to me.

t me back up a bit.

My grandparents were from Pittsburgh. One grandfather was a railroad worker who was electrocuted and killed on the job before I was born. The other grandfather was a miner and carpenter who had some craftiness in him. He died before I hit puberty from food poisoning complications and what would be summed up best as "natural causes". I don't think either of my grandmothers ever held jobs and they thought it was alien that my mom ended up being the first person in our family to go to college and become a teacher.

My dad worked with one of the many steel working companies in Cleveland as they were slowly getting bought up and turned into a monopoly. He suffered from a stroke when I was 5 and was completely incapable of working after that. He checked himself out of therapy and turned into a vegetable through his own lethargy. He has watched TV for the last 2o years or so and cannot walk by himself. He has very little communication ability, and has very few thoughts to communicate anyway.

I was an accident. My parents like to put it more politely that if they knew how much trouble one kid was they never would have had a second one. Knowing that my birth was unintentional it makes it a bit more sensitive that so many of my friends are having unplanned babies.

So when I was growing up we didn't have much money. We got social security and cu expenses. I had homemade clothes and haircuts done at home. We ate bland meals home 7 nights a week. I was sent to live with my grandmothers a few times. Those memories are kind of foggy but I always ended up back with my parents.

My friends from high school and I grew up on the far east side of Cleveland. My parents moved there because houses in the woods were cheap as shit. That was barely over thirty years ago and now it's a sterile suburb complete with strip malls, paranoia, and dysfunctional, repressed families.

The families we came from were no different.

It should be no surprise to anyone familiar with this kind of suburban environment that every one of my friends grew up in a house full of verbal, physical, mental, emotional, sexual, drug, or alcohol abuse. I think the most common combination was some of each. Many of the reasons that we were such close friends was due to what was going on in our homes. We created our own refuge in a park and would spend a good deal of time there.

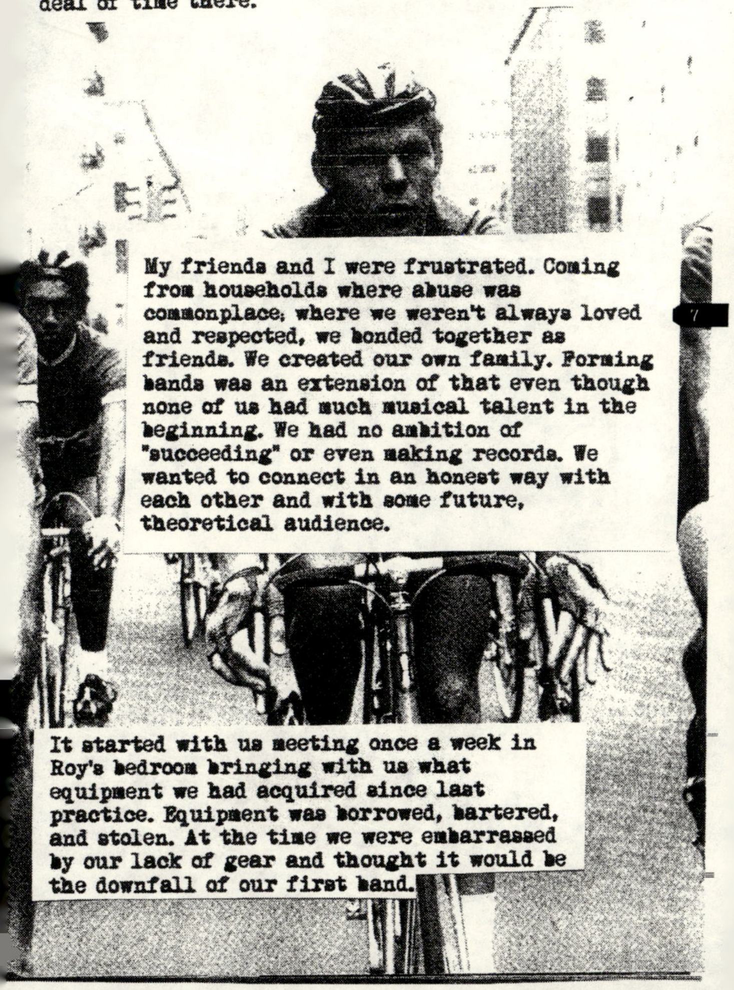

My friends and I were frustrated. Coming from households where abuse was commonplace; where we weren't always loved and respected, we bonded together as friends. We created our own family. Forming bands was an extension of that even though none of us had much musical talent in the beginning. We had no ambition of "succeeding" or even making records. We wanted to connect in an honest way with each other and with some future, theoretical audience.

It started with us meeting once a week in Roy's bedroom bringing with us what equipment we had acquired since last practice. Equipment was borrowed, bartered, and stolen. At the time we were embarrassed by our lack of gear and thought it would be the downfall of our first band.

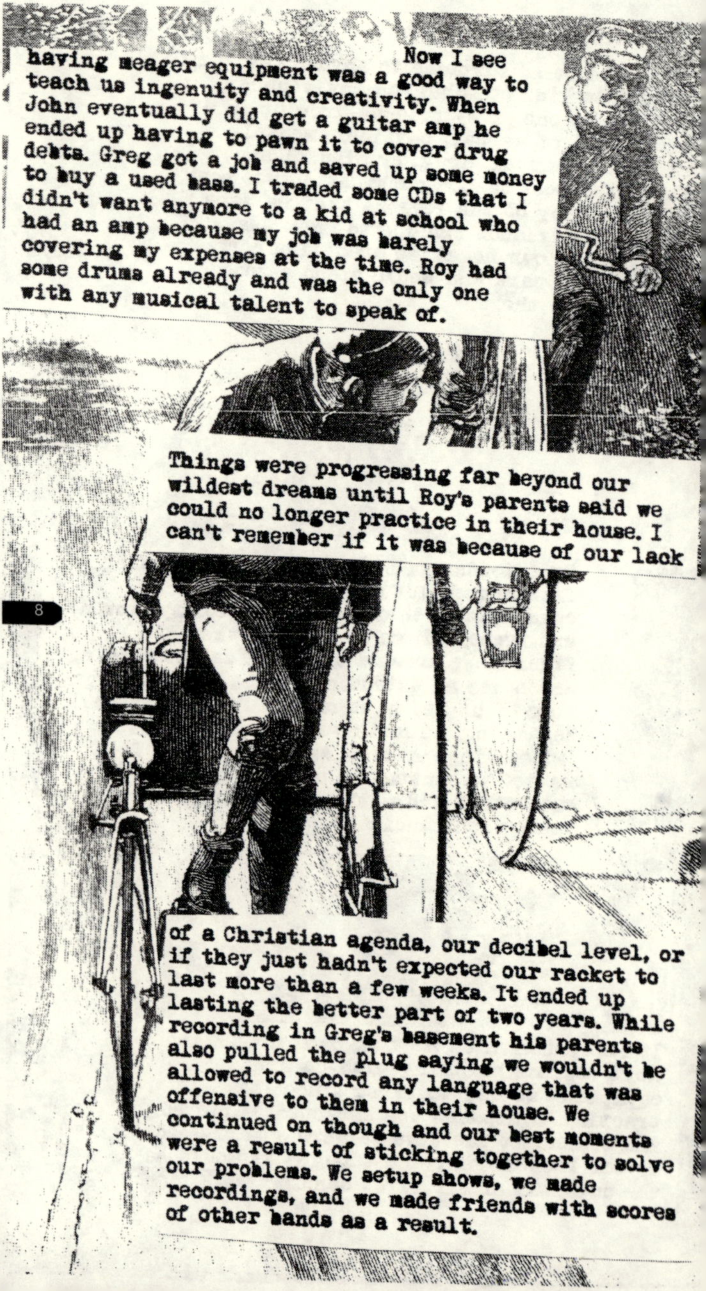

Now I see having meager equipment was a good way to teach us ingenuity and creativity. When John eventually did get a guitar amp he ended up having to pawn it to cover drug debts. Greg got a job and saved up some money to buy a used bass. I traded some CDs that I didn't want anymore to a kid at school who had an amp because my job was barely covering my expenses at the time. Roy had some drums already and was the only one with any musical talent to speak of.

Things were progressing far beyond our wildest dreams until Roy's parents said we could no longer practice in their house. I can't remember if it was because of our lack of a Christian agenda, our decibel level, or if they just hadn't expected our racket to last more than a few weeks. It ended up lasting the better part of two years. While recording in Greg's basement his parents also pulled the plug saying we wouldn't be allowed to record any language that was offensive to them in their house. We continued on though and our best moments were a result of sticking together to solve our problems. We setup shows, we made recordings, and we made friends with scores of other bands as a result.

ae end though, things fell apart as
often do. Everyone was a little upset
use I was playing in another band and
that it would hurt my schedule too
n. John wasn't always showing up for
ctice and his lack of work ethic was
ting on everyone's nerves. I think I got
ced before John was shown the door and
n things dissolved completely.

Sure, we got in fights (physical and verbal) but things worked out pretty well and we stuck by each other when we had problems, offering support and encouragement. We had our own family for awhile though and those bonds were too tough to sever. We took care of each other even outside of playing in our band together.

After everyone graduated from high school things started to change. I moved out and started supporting myself completely. John fell into a pretty bad cocaine habit. Roy went to college and started to try to take his future more seriously. Greg was working full time and living with me. I think he spent more time playing video games than anything else though. The most memorable moment was when he quit his job because a long awaited new game was released.

Fast forward a few years and it felt like everyone had abandoned their ethics. People thought it was strange and alien that I was still playing in bands and running a distro. They had moved on to careers or the scariest thought of all....having babies(!). I can't really remember who was the first to conceive a child but I remember that it struck me as odd. We were all kids raised in poor homes and I thought that at one point we had swore off becoming a mirror image of our parents.

We had all been in serious relationships i the past and I though we'd also become goo at behaving responsibly. I felt that up until that point we had all conquered som of our problems that we had learned from our parents. I was completely wrong.

It wouldn't have been such a big deal if having a baby was planned out and intentional but these babies were accidental; bred out of the same irresponsible nature that caused our parents to mistreat us. Maybe life was creating its circles twice as fast as we got older. John had a kid with a woman who was about 5 years older than him and married to someone else. Her and her husband were split up for good reasons but they could never afford the divorce so they were "separated". This caused the baby to legally belong to her husband as Ohio's laws are severely out of touch with the times. This particular incident was really hard to deal with because she had 3 other kids who were all neglected already and the new baby would inevitably just make all of it worse.

My friends and I rarely talked about sex as teenagers and I think part of that was the social stigma surrounding sex. The fact that we were all male would probably have caused the conversations to turn competitive, at least on some level. While I'm no saint, I've always made effort to use some sort of birth control because I knew I wasn't ready to be a parent. The prospects were quite scary to me and I've been very fortunate that I never had a faulty condem or other problematic situation.

Evelyn had a baby with a man that she barely knew who immediately left her when he found out she was pregnant. I think she expected the baby to make them closer but I doubt he even thinks about that kid too often while she is forced to be responsible for it everyday.

Another friend, Mary had a kid and quickly got married to the father. She later found out he was abusive and she eventually divorced him about a year later. Her daughter will never know her dad except through pictures.

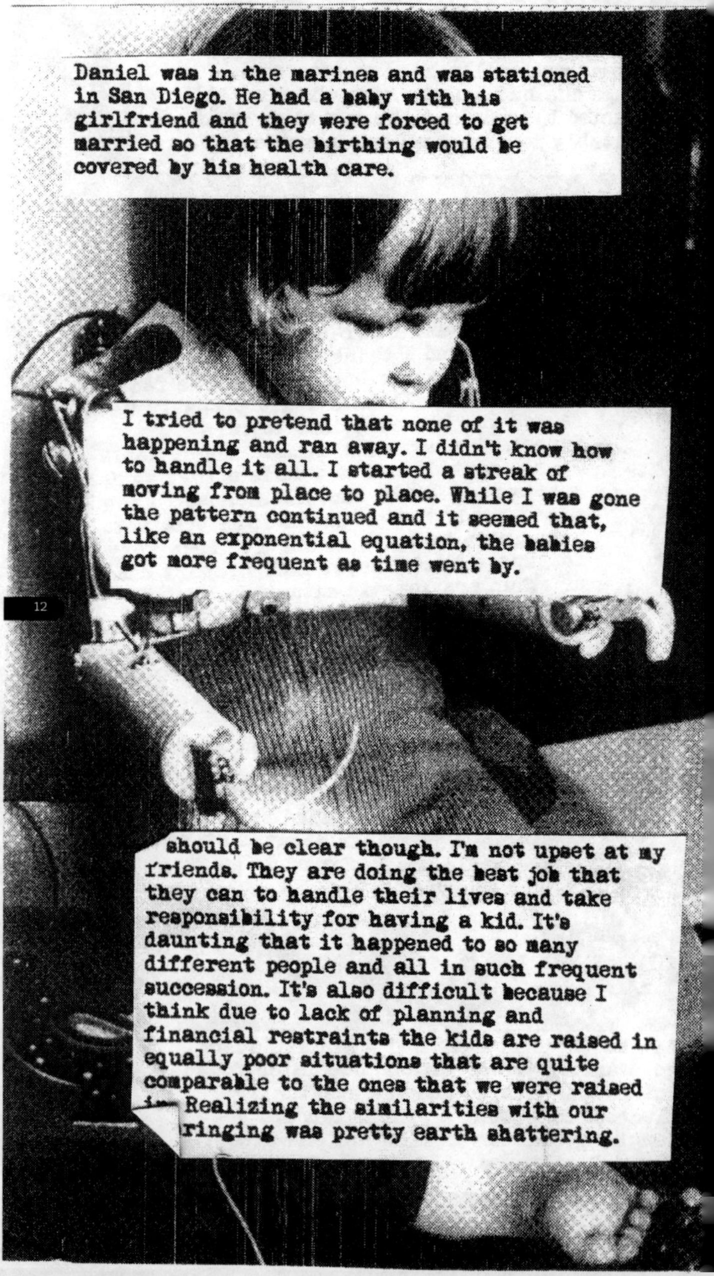

Daniel was in the marines and was stationed in San Diego. He had a baby with his girlfriend and they were forced to get married so that the birthing would be covered by his health care.

I tried to pretend that none of it was happening and ran away. I didn't know how to handle it all. I started a streak of moving from place to place. While I was gone the pattern continued and it seemed that, like an exponential equation, the babies got more frequent as time went by.

should be clear though. I'm not upset at my friends. They are doing the best job that they can to handle their lives and take responsibility for having a kid. It's daunting that it happened to so many different people and all in such frequent succession. It's also difficult because I think due to lack of planning and financial restraints the kids are raised in equally poor situations that are quite comparable to the ones that we were raised i[illegible] Realizing the similarities with our [illegible]ringing was pretty earth shattering.

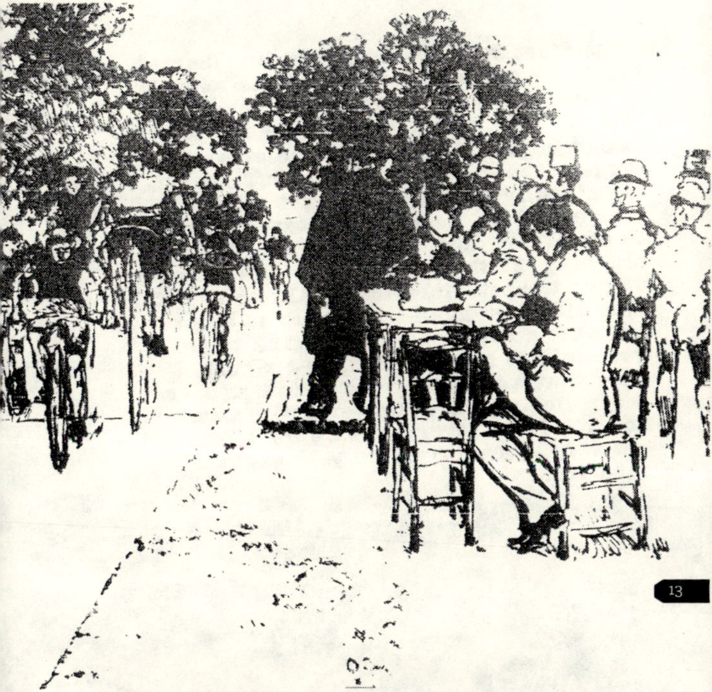

I've had friends who've had abortions and I felt that a great deal of my other friends would have been able to handle their lives better if they had not kept their babies through one means or another. Granted, that's not my place to tell them what to do with their lives but I'm certainly not opposed to the prospect for myself and relationships that I'm involved in. I've talked about it with partners recently and we've both come to terms that it's ultimately up to the woman and that I would be supportive in whatever ways were desired in the event that an abortion became necessary. Granted, these situations were theoretical and never needed acted upon but

it certainly helped our relationships to get these things talked about and out in the open.

I had first read about vasectomies, learned about the process involved and its benefits to other forms of contraception when I was 19. I was really intrigued. It was in Punk Planet Magazine, I think. A vasectomy is a surgery that involves cutting off the pipelines in your body that put sperm in your ejaculate. Basically it causes you to be sterile by closing off the proper plumbing. At that point I knew that I never wanted to have biological children and if I ever did have kids I would want to adopt and make a firm decision, knowing that I was ready to have a child. As a result, I knew that a vasectomy was something I was interested in and would seriously consider, however I had never had surgery before and was very squeamish where pain might be involved.

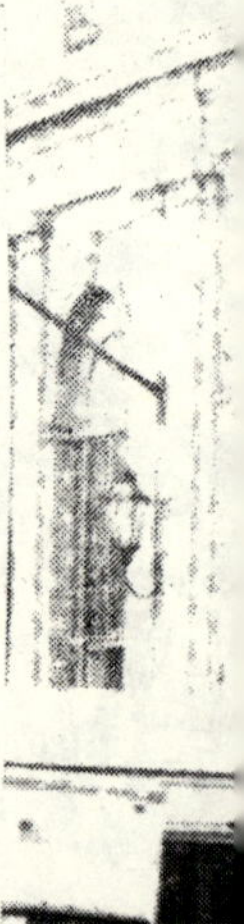

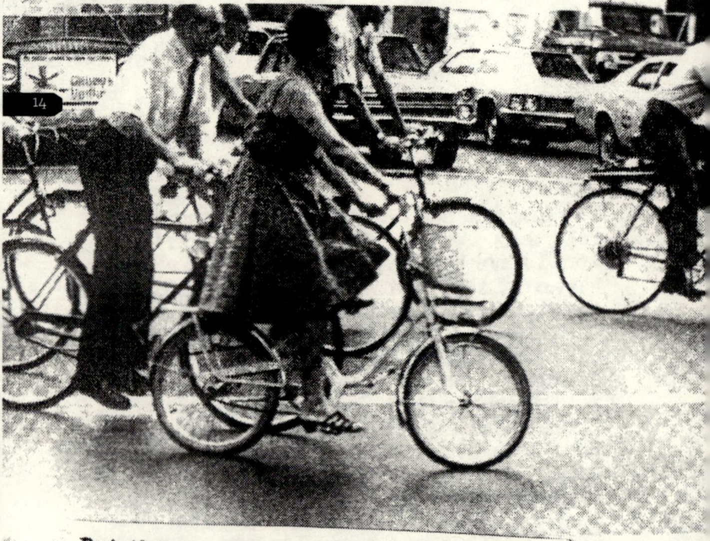

But this was serious. Did I want to turn into one of my friends with another accidental child that would convert my life to something less than the grand plans that I had laid out for myself? Hell no!

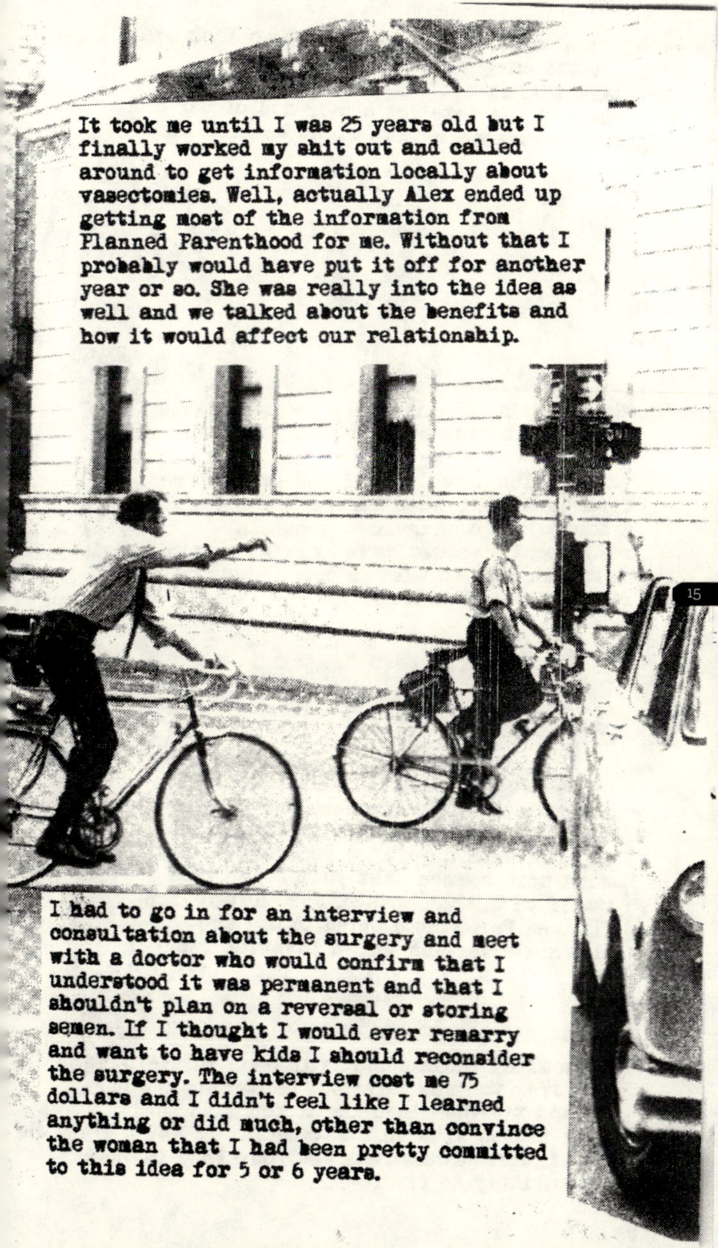

It took me until I was 25 years old but I finally worked my shit out and called around to get information locally about vasectomies. Well, actually Alex ended up getting most of the information from Planned Parenthood for me. Without that I probably would have put it off for another year or so. She was really into the idea as well and we talked about the benefits and how it would affect our relationship.

I had to go in for an interview and consultation about the surgery and meet with a doctor who would confirm that I understood it was permanent and that I shouldn't plan on a reversal or storing semen. If I thought I would ever remarry and want to have kids I should reconsider the surgery. The interview cost me 75 dollars and I didn't feel like I learned anything or did much, other than convince the woman that I had been pretty committed to this idea for 5 or 6 years.

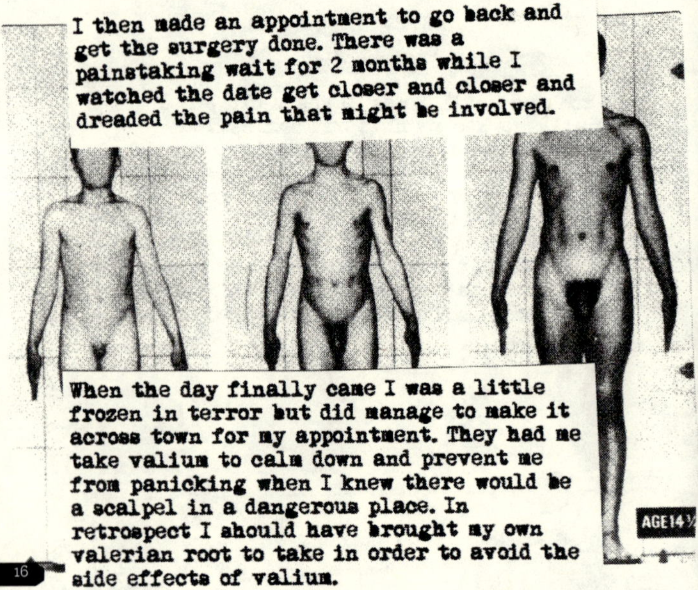

I then made an appointment to go back and get the surgery done. There was a painstaking wait for 2 months while I watched the date get closer and closer and dreaded the pain that might be involved.

When the day finally came I was a little frozen in terror but did manage to make it across town for my appointment. They had me take valium to calm down and prevent me from panicking when I knew there would be a scalpel in a dangerous place. In retrospect I should have brought my own valerian root to take in order to avoid the side effects of valium.

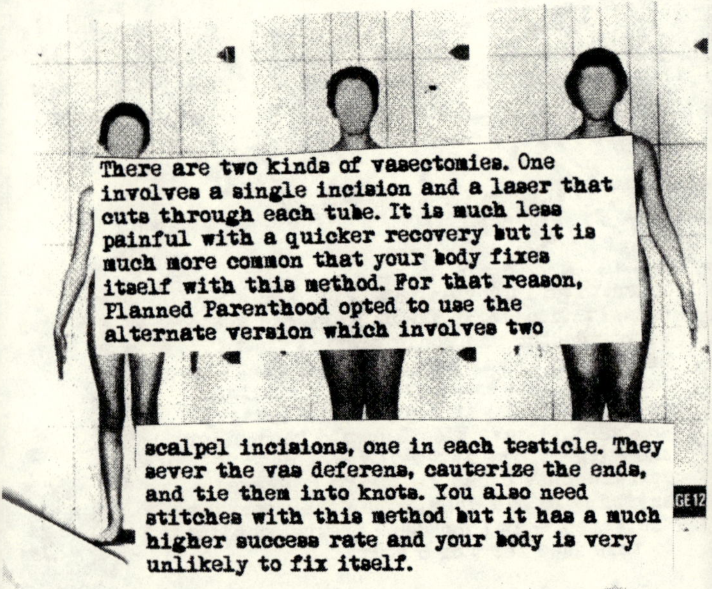

There are two kinds of vasectomies. One involves a single incision and a laser that cuts through each tube. It is much less painful with a quicker recovery but it is much more common that your body fixes itself with this method. For that reason, Planned Parenthood opted to use the alternate version which involves two scalpel incisions, one in each testicle. They sever the vas deferens, cauterize the ends, and tie them into knots. You also need stitches with this method but it has a much higher success rate and your body is very unlikely to fix itself.

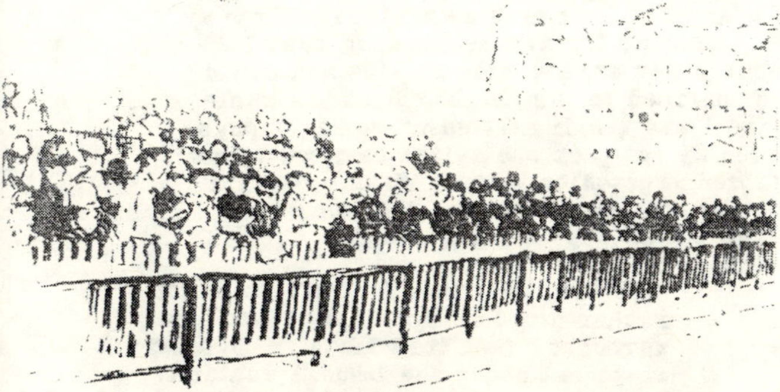

I sat down, prepared myself, and sat there in wait. It didn't seem like the valium was doing anything at first but I think that is because it's effect is to make you calm, not drugged - especially calm in the rare moment that people are poking sharp instruments into a sensitive part of your body. The surgery was really pretty easy considering all that was involved. I made jokes, asking the nurse if Christians came in to get vasectomies as a form of birth control. I thought it was funny but she wasn't amused and it turns out her family was Christian. The whole deal took about 20 minutes and I was back on my feet holding an icepack to my testicles and waddling back to the lobby.

I went home and sat on the couch for a few hours before going to bed. I slept for most of the weekend, waiting for the swelling to go down so I could begin to lead a normal life again. We had some Canadian house guests at the time and one of them was motivated enough to go and get a vasectomy of his own. That makes me feel like I'm succeeding at doing vasectomy outreach and education on some minute, personal level.

It took me about a week to get back into the swing of things and about two weeks before I started riding my bike again. That was my big hang up for awhile; knowing that I wouldn't be able to ride my bike and would be confined to our neighborhood the whole time I was healing. It wasn't so bad though. When my ice pack was melted we opted to use frozen vegetables instead. Everyone helped out by cooking for me and Alex made sure I always had everything I needed.

Now, with some time for reflection I'm rather proud of myself that I followed through. I feel that I have made a strong statement about the issue. I wouldn't demonize someone for having a child but I definitely feel that the world is overpopulated and it's our duty to do something about that. I commend radical parenting and the people who are capable of raising a child in that environment. At one time I would help take care of my friend Vicki's foster child and would pick her up from school and bond with her. It was truly magical and I felt like I was making a difference. However, it also required tons of patience and I would need time to relax later in the day. I don't think I am prepared to handle those kind of challenges full time at this point in my life.

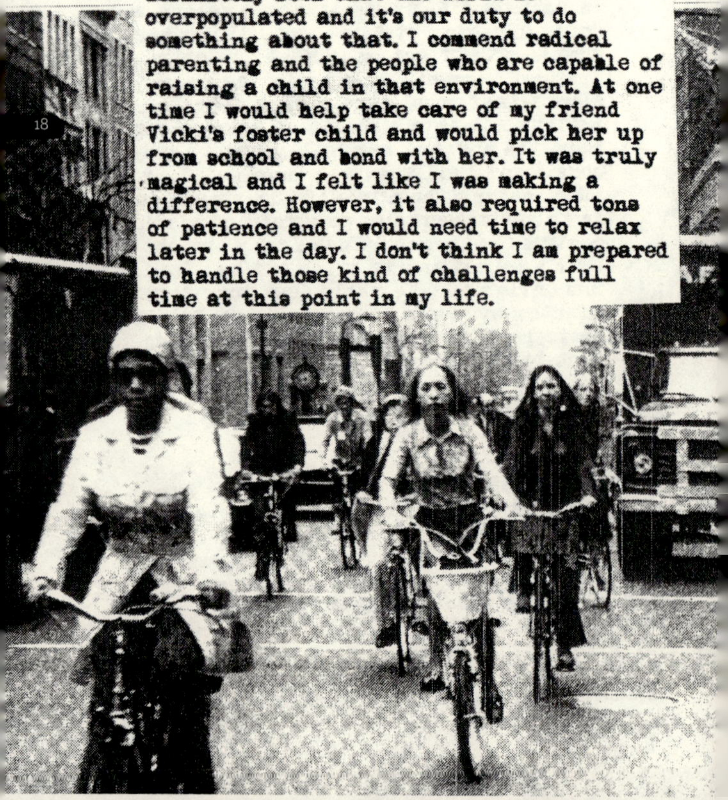

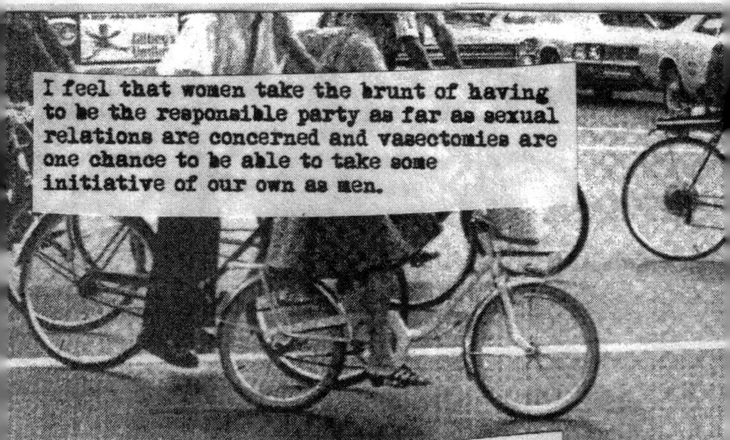

I feel that women take the brunt of having to be the responsible party as far as sexual relations are concerned and vasectomies are one chance to be able to take some initiative of our own as men.

Again, I'm not perfect and I've learned a lot about respecting women in the last 10 years but I've always tried to incorporate feminist values into my relationships. I see a lot of abuse towards women in other people's relationships and it pains me. I've been doing some house cleaning with my past relationships lately and calling people up that I haven't spoken to in years to re-evaluate the ways that I've treated them in the past.

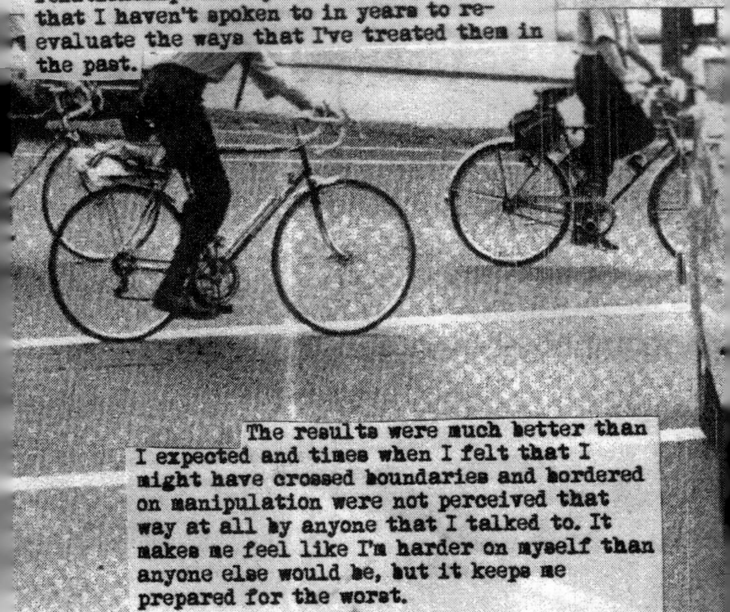

The results were much better than I expected and times when I felt that I might have crossed boundaries and bordered on manipulation were not perceived that way at all by anyone that I talked to. It makes me feel like I'm harder on myself than anyone else would be, but it keeps me prepared for the worst.

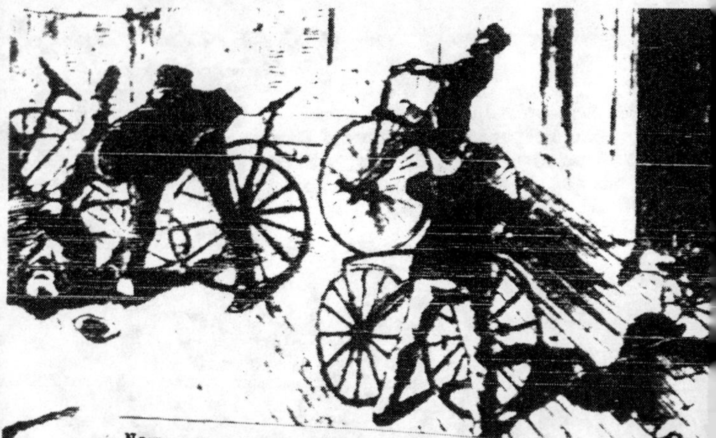

Now, many years later, my friends back home and I don't communicate as much or as often as we used to and I think part of that is because of our different life choices. When I tell people about my vasectomy it generally freaks them out and they can't understand why I would do that. I think it's pretty simple: I don't want to have biological children. We do all mutually respect each other and that's important but our values often get in the way during conversations because I sometimes forget that I live in the cultural ghetto of Portland where everyone is radical to varying degrees.

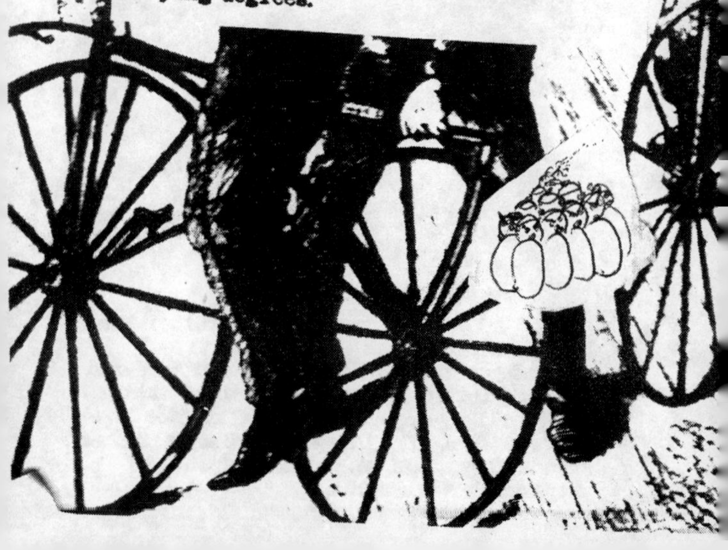

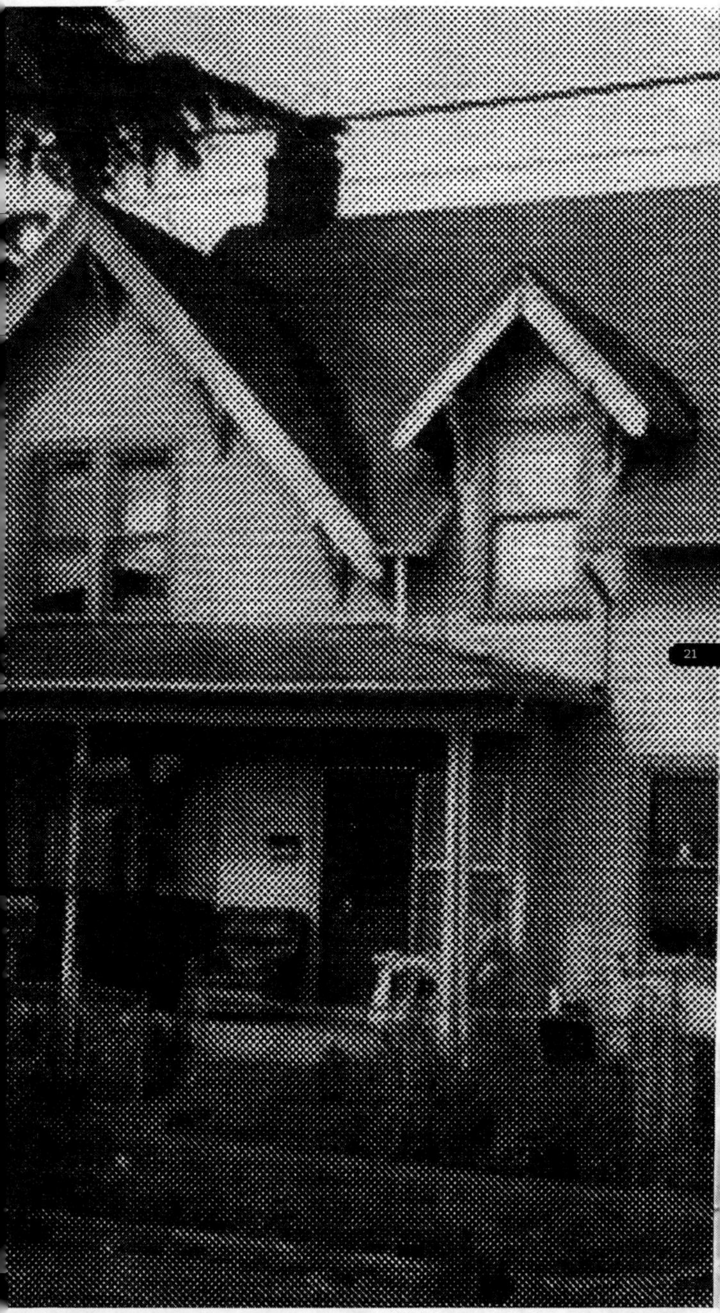

Roommate Reviews #4

In December of 2000 we finalized our deal to buy the house that we live in now. We had tons of problems finding the "right" roommates because we had just gotten out of a less-than-ideal living situation. We wanted people with similar values and expectations. We ended up hanging flyers and meeting with tons of people. The group that eventually moved in at first was Tim, Mell, Al, Sam, and Geoff.

Tim was the same germiphobe crusty punk that I had lived with in our last house and one of the few people who was on the same page with me...or so I thought. When he moved into this house he would constantly ridicule anyone who used the computer and intentionally do things that he knew would be annoyances to other people - like putting stencils around the house and criticizing people for being lazy. He would invite a dozen people over without telling anyone and hide things from people. Him and his girlfriend eventually had an accidental baby (conceived in our house!) and moved back to Minneapolis.

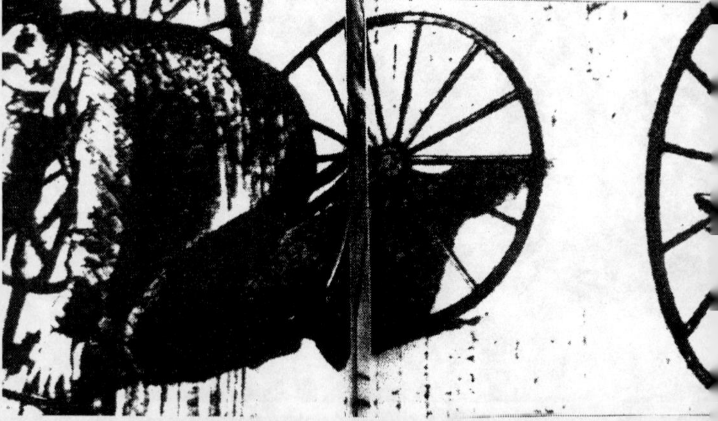

Al was a young idealistic kid just moving out of his parent's house. He had come to Portland on vacation a few times and had a pretty positive impression. Of course by the time he moved here he was stuck in a terrible relationship with someone who tormented him night and day. It fucked him up pretty bad and he quickly failed to do his dishes, clean up his messes, or do much of anything. Eventually he figured that the only way to get away from her manipulations was to move to Olympia and out of our house.

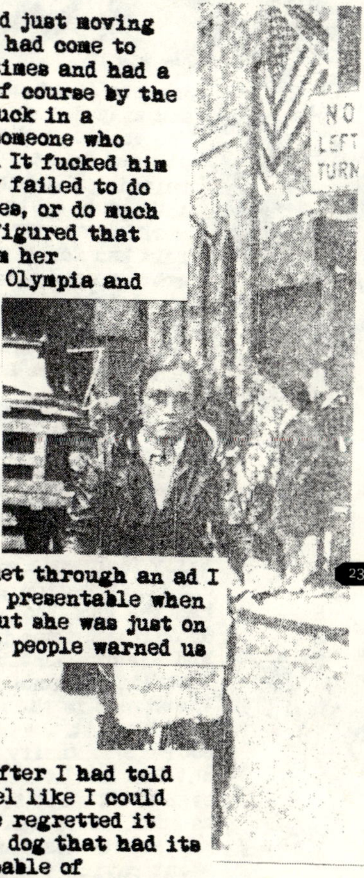

Mell was someone we had met through an ad I put up. She seemed rather presentable when we met her but it turns out she was just on her best behavior. Lots of people warned us about having her move in after I had told her it was okay. I didn't feel like I could revoke that decision and we regretted it bad. She had a trained show dog that had its bark removed and wasn't capable of socializing with people at all. Mell spent most of her nights at the bar, avoided house activities and responsibilities, owned a car but tried to convince us that she rarely used it, and talked about how much she enjoyed making zines and crafts. She would be passive aggressive in most conversations and would antagonize me for not going to every social function that was occurring. She moved out to go back to Seattle and tried to convince a few of our roommates to move out with her.

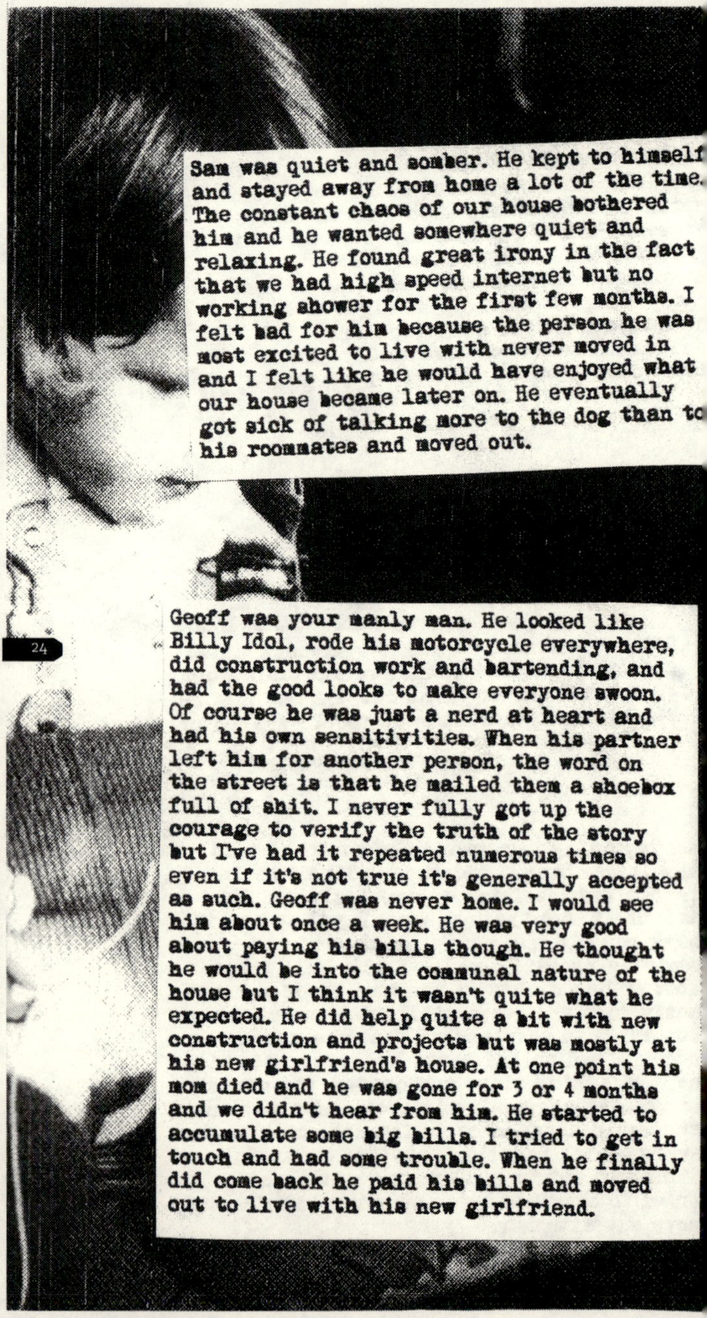

Sam was quiet and somber. He kept to himself and stayed away from home a lot of the time. The constant chaos of our house bothered him and he wanted somewhere quiet and relaxing. He found great irony in the fact that we had high speed internet but no working shower for the first few months. I felt bad for him because the person he was most excited to live with never moved in and I felt like he would have enjoyed what our house became later on. He eventually got sick of talking more to the dog than to his roommates and moved out.

Geoff was your manly man. He looked like Billy Idol, rode his motorcycle everywhere, did construction work and bartending, and had the good looks to make everyone swoon. Of course he was just a nerd at heart and had his own sensitivities. When his partner left him for another person, the word on the street is that he mailed them a shoebox full of shit. I never fully got up the courage to verify the truth of the story but I've had it repeated numerous times so even if it's not true it's generally accepted as such. Geoff was never home. I would see him about once a week. He was very good about paying his bills though. He thought he would be into the communal nature of the house but I think it wasn't quite what he expected. He did help quite a bit with new construction and projects but was mostly at his new girlfriend's house. At one point his mom died and he was gone for 3 or 4 months and we didn't hear from him. He started to accumulate some big bills. I tried to get in touch and had some trouble. When he finally did come back he paid his bills and moved out to live with his new girlfriend.

Please get in touch with reflections, thoughts, and
uestions.
Joe

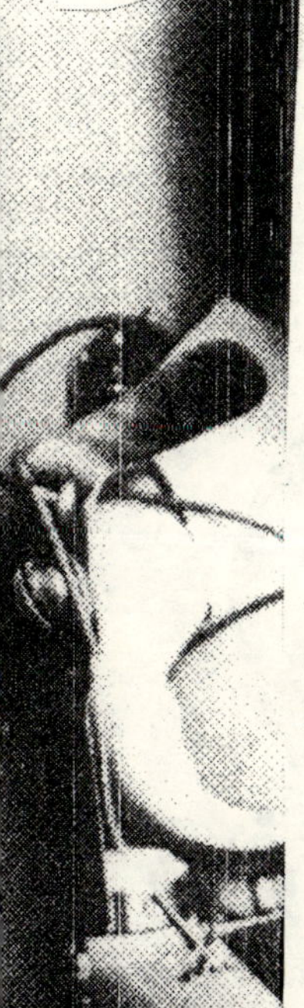

story by joe
edited by krissy,
eleanor, alex,
and britt
graphics from franco,
britt, and dustbin
dedicated to jason
for dealing with
shit that i never
could and keeping
true to his roots
made at the IPRC,
portland, or in 2004
write me. I hope to
get some good cookies
in trade.

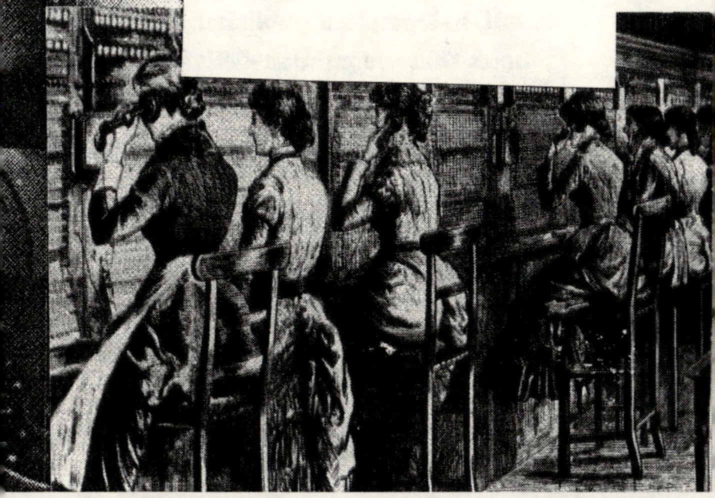

"more than rhetoric"
—Lunar Circuitry

"[Joe Biel previously] felt cont
to let other people articul
feelings...[Biel tells] stories
high school friends' inadvert
pregnancies and
[eventually ge
clipped at Plan
Parenthood. It's
pragma
that
think
of go
under
knif
—Zine T

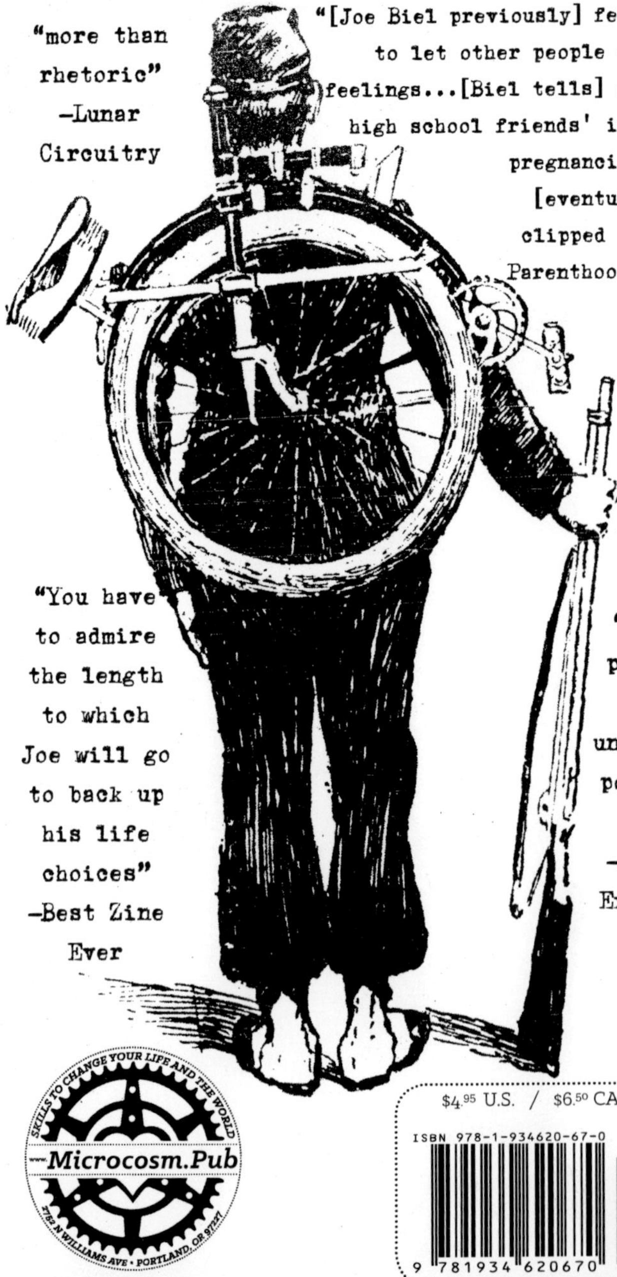

"You have to admire the length to which Joe will go to back up his life choices"
—Best Zine Ever

"Such a
persona
and
underlyi
politic
story"
—Profan
Existenc

SKILLS TO CHANGE YOUR LIFE AND THE WORLD
www.Microcosm.Pub
2752 N WILLIAMS AVE • PORTLAND, OR 97227

$4.95 U.S. / $6.50 CANADA

ISBN 978-1-934620-67-0
US$4.95
50495
9 781934 620670